THE

WEIGH
TO WIN
DAILY
JOURNAL

THE
WEIGH
TO WIN
DAILY
JOURNAL

LYNN HILL

FOUNDER OF WEIGH TO WIN, INC.

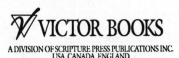

VICTOR BOOKS

A DIVISION OF SCRIPTURE PRESS PUBLICATIONS INC.
USA CANADA ENGLAND

All Scripture references are from the *Holy Bible, New International Version,* © 1973, 1978, 1984, International Bible Society. Used by permission of Zondervan Bible Publishers.

Editor: Greg D. Clouse

Cover Designer: Scott Rattray

ISBN No.: 0-89693-060-2

2 3 4 5 6 7 8 9 10 Printing/Year 96 95 94 93 92

To all the Weigh to Win *members and staff
who have been* my *inspiration through the years,
and with whom I rejoice that
"...nothing is impossible with God"
(Luke 1:37).*

How to Use This Journal

A quiet time with the Lord will help you gain perspective and strength from Him to carry you through the day ahead. Using this journal on a daily basis will also help you face the emotions which typically trigger problem-eating episodes in your life.

Overcoming the habits which have caused our weight problem is a battle that is not won overnight. Ecclesiastes 9:11 says, "The race is not to the swift or the battle to the strong." Willpower alone is not enough to win the battle. If it were, I would have lost the battle this time too. *Do not* expect God to make your choices for you, but *do* expect Him to be there when you call on Him for strength because He has promised, "Never will I leave you; never will I forsake you" (Hebrews 13:5).

For the next thirteen weeks you will begin your day by reading the letter which I have written for you at the start of each new week. In these letters I have shared from my experiences to give you hope and encouragement. As you reread the letter every day of your week, you will find the Lord revealing new insights as you dig deeper into the meaning of the words for your life. The Lord will give you a new perspective and strength through the daily reading of the accompanying Scripture. Then, study the testimonial or inspirational quotation written to give you encouragement on a daily basis and allow it to speak to your heart.

Start each day by writing down your feelings. Writing

helps you to confront your emotions and brings you one step closer to dealing with those feelings without turning to food. Allow yourself to *experience* the emotion as you write, without trying to push the emotion away with food. Cry if you need to. Feel your anger, frustration, resentment, disappointment, loneliness, or fear.

Hopefully, some of your emotions will be happy and joyful. Allow yourself to feel the joy, and recognize that happiness and food do not have to be forever linked together. You *can* be happy without food being an integral part of life's emotional experiences. Record these happy times in your journal. They will give you hope to get you through more difficult situations.

Next, write down a *positive* statement about yourself, your relationship with the Lord, your weight loss, your dreams, your plans, or your desires. Avoid negative thoughts which serve no purpose other than to pull you down to despair.

Take time to be silent. Give the Lord a chance to assure you of His love and care for you. He will reassure you of His presence in your daily life.

Use this journal as a tool to help you to succeed day by day, hour by hour, or minute by minute. Keep this journal with you where you can review the positive thought which you wrote for the day.

Finally, dear friend, I may not know you by name, but I do know your battle because it was and is my battle. I share your struggle. I hope to share the joy of your success.

"The Lord is my helper; I will not be afraid" (Hebrews 13:6).

LYNN HILL
Plymouth, Indiana

THE
WEIGH
TO WIN
DAILY
JOURNAL

Dear Friend in Christ,

The days, weeks, and months ahead are going to be the most difficult of your life. They are also going to be the most joy-filled. How can they be both?

Overeating is a habit and changing a lifelong habit is a most difficult accomplishment. Habits are cobwebs which turn into cables, and we have to unwrap that cable strand by strand. The cable of the overeating habit hurts us and is certainly not easy to carry around. Moving with this cable is heavy and awkward. Many of us have carried it around for so long that we are afraid to let go. We have become used to the hurt and pain.

However, gaining freedom from that cable (even strand by strand) means we are succeeding at accomplishing a goal. Every small step is full of joy as we replace the habit of making poor food choices with new, better food choices.

"The Lord lifts up those who are bowed down, the Lord loves the righteous. . . . Praise the Lord."
                                        (taken from Psalm 146)

Day 1

"Nineteen-eighty-two proved to be the year of my greatest despair. Nothing seemed to be working as Larry and I had planned. The family we had dreamed about together was not to be. I quit caring about anything, including myself and my appearance. I was carrying fifty pounds of extra weight on my five-feet one-inch frame. I was miserable inside and out.

"In January of 1989 my sister and I decided to attend the _Weigh to Win_ class in Winona Lake, Indiana. In just four short months I lost twenty-two pounds.

"I have stayed within five pounds of my desired weight now for one year and three months. I believe that with the help of God and _Weigh to Win,_ I will be able to keep that weight off indefinitely. Thank you, Lynn Hill! This new way of eating is something I can do for a lifetime!"

—_Beth_

_____

_____

_____

_____

_____

Day 2

When you are at the end of your rope, tie a knot and hang on.

_____

_____

_____

_____

_____

_____

_____

_____

_____

_____

Day 3

_____
Date

"Great is our Lord and mighty in power; His understanding has no limit" (Psalm 147:5).

_____

_____

_____

_____

_____

_____

_____

_____

_____

_____

_____

Day 4

Only "I" can change FAT to FIT.

_____

_____

_____

_____

_____

_____

_____

_____

_____

_____

_____

WEEK ONE
Day 5

_____
Date

"You give me Your shield of victory, and Your right hand sustains me" (Psalm 18:35).

_____

_____

_____

_____

_____

_____

_____

_____

_____

_____

Day 6

Date

Trouble is the common denominator of living. Do not wait until you do not have problems to begin changing your poor eating habits because that time never comes.

_____

_____

_____

_____

_____

_____

_____

_____

_____

_____

Day 7

Date

Dreams coming true begin with belief.

_____

_____

_____

_____

_____

_____

_____

_____

_____

_____

Dear Friend in Christ,

Do you find yourself making excuses?

"I can't follow this *Weigh to Win* Rainbow Food Plan because it has strawberries on it and I don't like strawberries."

"I can't start a weight loss program. My birthday is coming up in a month and I want to be able to eat cake and ice cream."

"If my spouse were just more supportive I could do it, but he/she keeps bringing home potato chips and I can't stay out of them."

"We always go out for pizza with our friends on Thursday night and I know I will eat too much, so I might as well not even start trying to lose weight."

You can make one excuse after another but you will just be delaying the real satisfaction of having control of your food choices. Take action! You do not have to eat certain foods or go to certain restaurants just because that's the way it has always been done. Ask your spouse to keep potato chips out of the house. Suggest to your friends that you eat at a restaurant where you know you can keep your eating within bounds. Your family and friends love you and they want the best for you. So speak up and stay in control!

"But they all alike began to make excuses" (Luke 14:18).

"Therefore, prepare your minds for action; be self-controlled" (1 Peter 1:13).

Day 1

"I have now lost twenty-five pounds in eight weeks. I have been fat all my life and would like to think I can be accepted as I am, for who I am, and NOT what I look like—but life just isn't that way. But, more important than what people think is what God thinks. While I realize I am gloriously and wonderfully made, I've also come to the point where I know it is up to me to take care of the body God has given me. I want nothing more than to lose this weight with God's help and to, in turn, give Him the glory. I cannot do it through my power but only through HIS.

"I have a long way to go and I become overwhelmed when I think about it. But God said He is "I AM," not I WAS or I WILL BE. I have learned to take my weight loss one pound at a time and not worry about how long it will take. I can do all things through Christ who strengthens me!"

—Cindy

Day 2

We may not be able to direct the wind, but we can adjust our sails.

_____

_____

_____

_____

_____

_____

_____

_____

_____

_____

Day 3

"Be joyful in hope, patient in affliction, faithful in prayer"
(Romans 12:12).

_____

_____

_____

_____

_____

_____

_____

_____

_____

_____

Day 4

A wish is a desire without an attempt.

_____

_____

_____

_____

_____

_____

_____

_____

_____

_____

_____

Day 5

Date

"Turn my eyes away from worthless things; renew my life according to Your Word" **(Psalm 119:37).**

_____

_____

_____

_____

_____

_____

_____

_____

_____

_____

_____

Day 6

_____

Go for results — not speed.

_____

_____

_____

_____

_____

_____

_____

_____

_____

_____

_____

Day 7

"He who heeds discipline shows the way to life"
(Proverbs 10:17).

_____

_____

_____

_____

_____

_____

_____

_____

_____

_____

_____

Dear Friend in Christ,

I walked into the restaurant and there stood one of those revolving glass cases full of dessert delicacies. Mile-high lemon meringue pie was being paraded in front of me in a never-ending visual enticement.

"O Lord," my heart cried. "I can just taste it!" My mouth watered and my hands began to shake as the inward battle of habit-versus-will raged. "After all, God, you put lemons, sugar cane, and eggs on this earth—why shouldn't I eat it?"

"Okay, Lord," I argued, "I will make You a bargain. I am going to go in this restaurant and eat a nice, sensible, healthy meal. By the time I finish the meal, I plan to be able to ignore that piece of pie, but right now I cannot see myself doing it without a burst of Your power."

By the time I had finished my baked chicken, baked potato, green beans, roll, and salad, my resolve was back. "I still want the pie, Lord, but I don't need the pie anymore."

"The Spirit of the Lord will come upon you in power . . . and you will be changed into a different person" (1 Samuel 10:6).

Day 1

"The only person I can change is me."
                              —Peg

_____

_____

_____

_____

_____

_____

_____

_____

_____

_____

Day 2

Date

Don't plan the future with a rearview mirror.

_____

_____

_____

_____

_____

_____

_____

_____

_____

_____

_____

Day 3

_____
Date

"I know what it is to be in need, and I know what it is to have plenty. I have learned the secret of being content in any and every situation, whether well fed or hungry, whether living in plenty or in want. I can do everything through Him who gives me strength" **(Philippians 4:12-13).**

_____

_____

_____

_____

_____

_____

_____

_____

_____

Day 4

_____
Date

A quitter never wins and a winner never quits.

_____

_____

_____

_____

_____

_____

_____

_____

_____

_____

Day 5

_____
Date

It isn't the mountains ahead that wear you out; it's the grain of sand in your shoe.

_____

_____

_____

_____

_____

_____

_____

_____

_____

_____

_____

Day 6

_____

"And my God will meet all your needs according to His glorious riches in Christ Jesus" (Philippians 4:19).

_____

_____

_____

_____

_____

_____

_____

_____

_____

_____

_____

Day 7

Date

Do not ask for more in your life without first saying "Thank You" for what you have already received.

_____

_____

_____

_____

_____

_____

_____

_____

_____

_____

Dear Friend in Christ,

My husband is at work, the children are in school, and I am
alone with the refrigerator. I have cleaned all the unhealthy
foods from the refrigerator and pantry, but I know that I can
binge on a box of saltine crackers and a chunk of cheese.

I hear the cheese calling my name from the refrigerator.
You see, my boss gave me an assignment at work which I
don't think I can handle. I feel overwhelmed. I just want to
drown my sorrows and fears in that chunk of cheese. I love
cheese so much that I should have been a mouse!

Turning on the television for distraction, an ice cream sundae with rivers of hot fudge fills the screen. I quickly turn off
the TV and start toward my bedroom to get a book. I stop
and catch a glimpse of myself in the mirror. No, I don't want
to look like this the rest of my life. I will have cheese and
crackers but only in the amounts I am allowed.

> *"The wisdom of the prudent is to give thought to their ways,
> but the folly of fools is deception"* *(Proverbs 14:8).*

Day 1

_____
Date

"I have tried many other diets without success. I decided to try the *Weigh to Win* system as a last resort. I have lost seventy-two pounds on the *Weigh to Win* Rainbow Food Plan. I eat more food than on any other program and still lose weight. My husband eats the same way I do and likes the food. I could not have done it without God's help and our support group leader who is the inspiration of the group."

—Norma

_____

_____

_____

_____

_____

_____

_____

_____

Day 2

Break the pattern and go for steadfast progress instead of flashes of brilliance.

_____

_____

_____

_____

_____

_____

_____

_____

_____

_____

_____

Day 3

Date

"Let us run with perseverance the race marked out for us"
(Hebrews 12:1).

_____

_____

_____

_____

_____

_____

_____

_____

_____

_____

Day 4

There are four tools needed to reach your goal: determination, dedication, discipline, and most important, attitude.

_____

_____

_____

_____

_____

_____

_____

_____

_____

_____

_____

Day 5

"I will not sacrifice to the Lord my God . . . offerings that cost me nothing" (2 Samuel 24:24).

Everything worthwhile has a price to be paid for it. What are you offering to the Lord? What is it costing you? Are you presenting your offering with an attitude of joy?

_____

_____

_____

_____

_____

_____

_____

_____

_____

Day 6

_____
Date

We only fail when we give up trying.

_____

_____

_____

_____

_____

_____

_____

_____

_____

_____

Day 7

Date

"With Your help I can advance against a troop; with my God I can scale a wall" (2 Samuel 22:30).

_____

_____

_____

_____

_____

_____

_____

_____

_____

_____

Dear Friend in Christ,

Overeating and making poor food choices is a learned response to life events. It is not a spiritual problem.

As a child, my family moved almost every year. Mom and I would bury our loneliness and apprehension by baking a batch of cookies. Actually, we never baked "a" batch—it was always a quadruple batch and they were gone within a day or two. When I would fall down and skin my knee, I was handed a piece of candy with, "Here, this will make it feel better!" When I went to the doctor's office and got a shot, I received a sucker as a reward for enduring the pain somewhat courageously. Consequently, I learned that food was the answer for when I was hurting, lonely, or depressed.

Times of celebration always seem to be centered around food. Doing something "as a family" meant going out to eat. A good report card meant a trip to the ice cream shop for a treat. Consequently, I learned to associate food with feeling good or happy.

If you stop to think about it, we are usually happy or sad for some reason. Seldom do we start the day by saying, "I feel indifferent today." If we have learned that food is the answer for sad times and that it is the answer for happy times, then food becomes the answer for all of life's emotions and events.

Eating for emotional reasons becomes a habit and is so ingrained that it takes more than willpower to succeed. We need the Lord's help to be an overcomer!

"Who is it that overcomes the world? Only he who believes that Jesus is the Son of God" (1 John 5:5).

Day 1

"I have tried many diet programs in the last eighteen years and have always gained back the weight. I have been on the *Weigh to Win* system for one month and have lost eleven pounds. I wake up in the morning and I feel good that I am doing something for myself. I don't feel guilty when I eat, because it's healthy, it's good, and I'm losing weight. I have more self-esteem and energy too.

"The main reason I believe that *Weigh to Win* works over other programs is because it meets both your spiritual and physical needs—and that is a winning combination!

"My favorite Scripture that helps me daily is, 'The joy of the Lord is your [my] strength' " (Nehemiah 8:10).

—Kris

_____

_____

_____

_____

_____

_____

Day 2

Prior planning prevents poor performance.

_____

_____

_____

_____

_____

_____

_____

_____

_____

_____

_____

Day 3

"Set your minds on things above, not on earthly things"
(Colossians 3:2).

_____

_____

_____

_____

_____

_____

_____

_____

_____

_____

_____

Day 4

It is no disgrace to start over—it is usually an opportunity.

_____

_____

_____

_____

_____

_____

_____

_____

_____

_____

Day 5

"If you always do what you've always done, you'll always get what you always got and you'll always be what you've always been."

Are you lapsing back into some old eating habits? If so, what are you going to do about it? If not, write a thank you note to the Lord and give yourself a pat on the back!

_____

_____

_____

_____

_____

_____

_____

_____

Day 6

"Do not be anxious about anything, but in everything, by prayer and petition, with thanksgiving, present your requests to God. And the peace of God, which transcends all understanding, will guard your hearts and your minds in Christ Jesus" (Philippians 4:6-7).

_____

_____

_____

_____

_____

_____

_____

_____

_____

_____

Day 7

_____
Date

Triumph is "try" with a lot of "umph."

_____

_____

_____

_____

_____

_____

_____

_____

_____

_____

_____

WEEK SIX

Dear Friend in Christ,

The alarm just went off at five-thirty in the morning. I have my walking shoes and sweatsuit laid out next to the bed to eliminate the excuse of not being able to find my shoes or clothes.

"Lord," I argued, "why can't I just be naturally skinny and beautiful like my size six sister-in-law? She doesn't get up at five-thirty in the morning to walk off *her* body fat," I whined.

"Quit arguing and get out there," God spoke in a firm but loving voice. "I did give you a beautiful body but you did not care for it properly, so now you have to work to get it back in shape. Now get out there and walk and pray and we will fellowship together."

"Okay, God—I'm on my way!"

"Don't have anything to do with foolish and stupid arguments, because you know they produce quarrels. And the Lord's servant must not quarrel; instead, he must be kind to everyone ... not resentful" (2 Timothy 2:23-24).

Day 1

There are thousands to tell you it cannot be done,
There are thousands to prophesy failure;
There are thousands to point out to you one by one,
The dangers that wait to assail you.
But just buckle in with a bit of a grin;
Just take off your coat and go to it;
Just start in to sing as you tackle the thing
That "cannot be done," and you'll do it.

—*Edgar A. Guest*

_____

_____

_____

_____

_____

_____

_____

_____

Day 2

_____

"Therefore I tell you, do not worry about your life, what you will eat or drink; or about your body, what you will wear. Is not life more important than food, and the body more important than clothes?" **(Matthew 6:25)**

_____

_____

_____

_____

_____

_____

_____

_____

_____

_____

Day 3

Date

The road to success is marked with many tempting parking places. Don't take advantage of them or you will never reach the end of your journey!

_____

_____

_____

_____

_____

_____

_____

_____

_____

_____

Day 4

Date

"But if it were I, I would appeal to God; I would lay my cause before Him. He performs wonders that cannot be fathomed, miracles that cannot be counted" **(Job 5:8-9).**

_____

_____

_____

_____

_____

_____

_____

_____

_____

_____

Day 5

_____
Date

Without commitment, your automatic response is to avoid difficulties. Are you committed to the changes you must make in your life in order to take care of your body from the inside out?

_____

_____

_____

_____

_____

_____

_____

_____

_____

_____

_____

Day 6

_____

"Teach me, and I will be quiet; show me where I have been wrong. How painful are honest words!"
(Job 6:24-25)

_____

_____

_____

_____

_____

_____

_____

_____

_____

Day 7

Some people grin and bear it. Successful people smile and change it. What do you need to "smile and change" in your life?

_____

_____

_____

_____

_____

_____

_____

_____

_____

_____

Dear Friend in Christ,

Everyone wants to lose weight FAST. There are a myriad of advertisements on television and in the newspapers which promise a "quick and easy" weight loss. I know this to be true because I have been persuaded to try many of them only to disappointedly discover that it also was "quick and easy" to put the weight right back on!

With the *Weigh to Win Weight Management System,* the average weight loss is one-half to two pounds per week. *Weigh to Win* does not promise you a faster weight loss because to lose weight more quickly may mean depriving your body of essential nutrients. A slow, safe weight loss means a greater percentage of fat is used by the body and there is less loss of important lean muscle tissue. Besides, you did not gain your weight overnight and it is not going to disappear overnight.

Throughout my weight loss journey, people would often ask how much more weight I was going to lose. When you have as much weight to lose as I had, it can be very discouraging to look down the road at how far you have to go to reach your goal. Instead of allowing myself to become discouraged at this prospect, I would answer their question with, "I don't know how far I have to go, but so far I have lost ____ pounds!"

Do not focus on how long your journey will take. Concentrate on how far you have come and build on that success.

"For this reason, since the day we heard about you, we have not stopped praying for you and asking God to fill you with the knowledge of His will through all spiritual wisdom and understanding. And we pray this in order that you may live a life worthy of the Lord and may please Him in every way: bearing fruit in every good work, growing in the knowledge of God, being strengthened with all power according to His glorious might so that you may have great endurance and patience, and joyfully giving thanks to the Father, who has qualified you to share in the inheritance of the saints in the kingdom of light" (Colossians 1:9-12, emphasis added).

Whether you have just a few pounds to lose or many, your journey is a lifelong one as you work to permanently change poor eating habits. Pray for "endurance and patience" as you take one day at a time on your road to success.

Day 1

"I believe in *Weigh to Win,* not only because the system is the best there is, but I believe in what *Weigh to Win* stands for. *Weigh to Win's* emphasis that God is our Leader, our Strength, and the One who sees us through has been the key to success for me and many others.

"I have lost twenty-five pounds on the *Weigh to Win* system. I did not lose weight at first because I did not have my mind set on my goal. I guess I just did not want to lose weight badly enough. But once I made up my mind that I wanted to lose weight for my sake, and was faithful to the *Weigh to Win* Rainbow Food Plan, my perseverance paid off. If you are faithful to the *Weigh to Win* Rainbow Food Plan, it will be faithful to you too."

— *Sandie*

Day 2

Date

"The Lord has done great things for us, and we are filled with joy" (Psalm 126:3).

_____

_____

_____

_____

_____

_____

_____

_____

_____

_____

_____

Day 3

_____
Date

Focus on the benefits, not the activity.

_____

_____

_____

_____

_____

_____

_____

_____

_____

_____

Day 4

Date

"*But thanks be to God! He gives us the victory through our Lord Jesus Christ. Therefore, my dear brothers, stand firm. Let nothing move you*" *(1 Corinthians 15:57-58).*

_____

_____

_____

_____

_____

_____

_____

_____

_____

_____

Day 5

_____

Your belief at the beginning of a doubtful undertaking is the one thing that ensures the successful outcome of your venture.

_____

_____

_____

_____

_____

_____

_____

_____

_____

_____

Day 6

"But He said to them, 'I have food to eat that you know nothing about.'

"Then His disciples said to each other, 'Could someone have brought Him food?'

" 'My food,' said Jesus, 'is to do the will of Him who sent Me and to finish His work' " (John 4:32-34).

_____

_____

_____

_____

_____

_____

_____

_____

_____

_____

Day 7

Many overweight persons are victims of negative thinking because they have failed so often. This is the first thing to change. Positive thinkers get powerful results.

_____

_____

_____

_____

_____

_____

_____

_____

_____

_____

Dear Friend in Christ,

Most of my life I have been on some type of weight loss program or special diet. I used to say that if I was not at least trying, I would weigh a ton! Each time I would try, I refused to face the reality that, yes, I would lose thirty to forty pounds, but then I would gain back fifty as soon as I quit the diet.

My weight was going up and up. Sure, it was only about ten pounds a year, but in ten years that adds up to 100 pounds!

What helped me to be successful with my weight loss this time was realizing that a diet was not what I needed. A diet implies something you that "go on" and "go off" of. I need-ed a plan which I could follow for the rest of my life. The *Weigh to Win* Rainbow Food Plan gave me the road map, but I had to take the journey.

For years I had prayed and asked God to take away my desire to overeat or to keep me from being tempted by foods which were not healthy choices. I have since learned that God is not going to take a hot fudge sundae out of my hands if I choose to eat it. However, if I tell Him that I *want* to resist food which would not be healthy for my body but I need Him to give me the strength to do it, then He is there to help me. Do you see the difference?

"Resist the devil, and he will flee from you. Come near to God and He will come near to you" (James 4:7-8).

WEEK EIGHT
Day 1

_____
Date

"It is surprising to realize that three quarters of the year have passed since beginning the *Weigh to Win* group at our church, supporting the saying, 'Time flies when you are having fun.'

"Sharing the oral presentation of the weekly lesson with other members of the group, I have found the 'blessing' of accountability. With the many diets I've tried, I honestly had little faith in one more. The remaining effect of my Yo-Yo style of weight control always left me twenty pounds plus from any goal weight. Those pounds became my protective package which kept me from confronting the issues causing my eating problem.

"With *Weigh to Win* I am having an average weight loss of one-quarter pound per week. Answering prayer, God is gently making me aware, turning me to honestly face responsibility, and teaching me not to give up and quit."

—Rita

_____

_____

_____

_____

Day 2

Date

To accomplish great things, we must not only act, but also dream, not only plan, but also believe.

_____

_____

_____

_____

_____

_____

_____

_____

_____

_____

Day 3

Date

"Trust in the Lord with all your heart and lean not on your own understanding; in all your ways acknowledge Him, and He will make your paths straight" **(Proverbs 3:5-6).**

_____

_____

_____

_____

_____

_____

_____

_____

_____

_____

WEEK EIGHT

Day 4

Date

Trying to lose weight your way has not worked. So, follow the Weigh to Win Weight Management System. It is tried and true and—it works!

_____

_____

_____

_____

_____

_____

_____

_____

_____

_____

78

Day 5

"Do not conform any longer to the pattern of this world, but be transformed by the renewing of your mind. Then you will be able to test and approve what God's will is—His good, pleasing and perfect will" **(Romans 12:2).**

_____

_____

_____

_____

_____

_____

_____

_____

_____

_____

Day 6

Success is overcoming your handicaps, your barriers, and your obstacles.

_____

_____

_____

_____

_____

_____

_____

_____

_____

_____

Day 7

_____
Date

"Love your neighbor as yourself" **(Romans 13:9).**

_____

_____

_____

_____

_____

_____

_____

_____

_____

_____

WEEK NINE

Dear Friend in Christ,

Through my year-long weight loss journey and the years since, my husband has worked for a bakery. We used to keep every kind of snack cake, Danish, pie, or cookie you can imagine available at an arm's reach.

At first, not fully realizing that too much of these foods were not healthy for my family, and not wanting to "deprive" my family of "their" treats just because I was trying to lose weight, I decided that I would just have to be strong and resist the tempting foods which surrounded me.

Three days into my weight loss program I found myself three bites into a caramel-and-pecan Danish. A small, quiet voice from within (or was it from above?) said, "Lynn, what are you doing?" I had not even realized what I was doing! I do not even remember unwrapping the Danish, and I had not even tasted what I had eaten. But, there it was, the gooey mess in my hand—evidence of my pending failure. I said to myself, "All right, Lynn, this is a test. Satan would like nothing more than to use this incident to prove that you are a failure and cause you to give up on losing weight. Will you

83

pass or fail?" I walked to the wastebasket with my hands shaking because I had been taught to not waste food—and threw away the Danish.

"Search me, O God, and know my heart; test me and know my anxious thoughts" (Psalm 139:23).

Day 1

_____

"To me, _Weigh to Win_ was a gift from God."
—_Janet (lost 113 pounds)_

_____

_____

_____

_____

_____

_____

_____

_____

_____

_____

Day 2

"When my spirit grows faint within me, it is You who know my way" (Psalm 142:3).

_____

_____

_____

_____

_____

_____

_____

_____

_____

_____

_____

_____

Day 3

Use whatever means it takes to get you through a successful day. Success breeds success. Each successful day makes you stronger for the next day. Just work on each individual day. Do not try to take on the whole world—it is just too overwhelming!

_____

_____

_____

_____

_____

_____

_____

_____

WEEK NINE
Day 4

Date

"Peace I leave with you; My peace I give you. I do not give to you as the world gives. Do not let your hearts be troubled and do not be afraid" (John 14:27).

_____

_____

_____

_____

_____

_____

_____

_____

_____

88

Day 5

_____
Date

Remember the sunshine when the storm seems unending.

_____

_____

_____

_____

_____

_____

_____

_____

_____

_____

Day 6

_____
Date

"The Lord is the stronghold of my life — of whom shall I be afraid?" (Psalm 27:1)

_____

_____

_____

_____

_____

_____

_____

_____

_____

_____

_____

Day 7

Date

Do not expect perfection in all that you do, but pray for wisdom not to repeat mistakes.

_____

_____

_____

_____

_____

_____

_____

_____

_____

_____

_____

Dear Friend in Christ,

I know the Lord loves me just as I am. He knows that I love Him too. The Bible even says that He created me in His image, but, oh, what I did with the body He created! Sure, much of the way I looked was from eating habits I had learned from childhood on, but it was time to take responsibility for my own actions and do something about it.

We seldom just stop a bad habit—we have to replace it with a good one. I did not want to give up pies and desserts and casseroles, but I found out that I did not have to. I learned how to make the most delicious dishes using little or no fat and little or no sugar. My family even loved them!

Now I can truly eat deliciously without a twinge of guilt because I know that what I eat is going to give me and my family a better, healthier life.

> *"Go, eat your food with gladness, and drink your wine with a joyful heart, for it is now that God favors what you do"* *(Ecclesiastes 9:7).*

Day 1

"Ultimately, we must call on God for solutions. His purposes are wiser than ours. Excessive worry only increases the problems, whereas prayer and thanksgiving to God, for help in solving problems, often lead to surprising solutions."
                                          —*John Marks Templeton*

Day 2

Make fitness a focus of your life.

_____

_____

_____

_____

_____

_____

_____

_____

_____

_____

Day 3

"The Lord does not look at the things man looks at. Man looks at the outward appearance, but the Lord looks at the heart" *(1 Samuel 16:7).*

_____

_____

_____

_____

_____

_____

_____

_____

_____

_____

Day 4

_____
Date

There are lessons to be learned in everything we experience. Never be afraid to try something new for it is from new experiences that we continue to grow.

_____

_____

_____

_____

_____

_____

_____

_____

_____

_____

Day 5

_____

"At the end of your life you will groan, when your flesh and body are spent. You will say, 'How I hated discipline! How my heart spurned correction! I would not obey my teachers or listen to my instructors'" **(Proverbs 5:11-13).**

Are you disciplined about completing your *Weigh to Win* Weekly Food Records?

_____

_____

_____

_____

_____

_____

_____

_____

Day 6

_____

When you are busy doing God's will, it is always too soon to quit.

_____

_____

_____

_____

_____

_____

_____

_____

_____

_____

"Ask and it will be given you; seek and you will find; knock and the door will be opened to you. For everyone who asks receives; he who seeks finds; and to him who knocks, the door will be opened" (Matthew 7:7-8).

_____

_____

_____

_____

_____

_____

_____

_____

_____

Dear Friend in Christ,

Have you ever watched how some thin people eat pizza? They leave the crust. They also just eat the filling out of pumpkin pie and leave the tender, flaky crust. They sit and push their food around on their plates with their forks as if they had nothing better to do with it. They never look to see how many pieces the cake has been cut into to be sure they get their fair share, and they don't consider it a "reward" to get the piece with the icing rose. Food just is not important to them. Being with friends and enjoying the fellowship of others is more important. Of course, there are exceptions, but these are "thin eating behaviors."

I knew that if I was going to keep my weight off, I would have to imitate these "thin eating behaviors." I practiced leaving a green bean on my plate just to be sure I had control over the must-clean-your-plate habit. When thinking about who I was going to be able to talk to at the church picnic became my focus instead of sister Alice's famous Dutch apple pie—I knew that I was making progress.

"Be imitators of God, therefore, as dearly loved children and live a life of love, just as Christ loved us and gave Himself up for us as a fragrant offering and sacrifice to God" (Ephesians 5:1-2).

Day 1

Date

"I have been a member of *Weigh to Win* for eight weeks and have lost twenty and one-half pounds. The food plan is great. What is so nice about it is that you use real food and the family can eat right along with you. My husband is a diabetic and the Rainbow Food Plan is good for him also. My motto is, 'I have a choice.' I also like the saying, 'Do your don't.' I have made the choice to 'do' and I am beginning to see the results. With God's help I *will* make my goal."

—Burl

Day 2

_____
Date

"Then you will call, and the Lord will answer; you will cry for help, and He will say: Here am I" (Isaiah 58:9).

_____

_____

_____

_____

_____

_____

_____

_____

_____

_____

_____

Day 3

_____

"Nothing is so full of victory as patience. He that can have patience can have what he will."

—*Ben Franklin*

_____

_____

_____

_____

_____

_____

_____

_____

_____

_____

Day 4

"Love . . . rejoices with the truth. It always protects, always trusts, always hopes, always perseveres. Love never fails" **(1 Corinthians 13:6-8).**

_____

_____

_____

_____

_____

_____

_____

_____

_____

_____

Day 5

_____

The best preparation for tomorrow is the proper use of today.

_____

_____

_____

_____

_____

_____

_____

_____

_____

_____

_____

"Teach me to do Your will, for You are my God; may Your good Spirit lead me on level ground" (Psalm 143:10).

_____

_____

_____

_____

_____

_____

_____

_____

_____

_____

Day 7

_____
Date

Dreams are goals with deadlines.

_____

_____

_____

_____

_____

_____

_____

_____

_____

_____

Dear Friend in Christ,

Do I ever make poor food choices? Sure, I make mistakes sometimes. After all, I was overweight longer than I have been thin, and sometimes it is just more comfortable to return to those old habits instead of staying with these new habits God and I are developing. However, I have learned that even when I stumble, it is easy to get back on the right path. When I make a poor choice, I just don't feel as good as when I am eating right.

Sometimes when I stumble, Satan, the deceiver, taunts me with, "See, I knew you couldn't do it—you are going to fail again." But I have learned to recognize him for what he is. I refuse to allow him to make me feel guilty and rob me of the love I know the Lord has for me. I refuse to let him rob me of my self-esteem. I refuse to let him rob me of success.

If I stumble, I just have to accept it as a detour on my journey to health and fitness, put it in the past (but learn from it), and then get right back on the *Weigh to Win* Rainbow Food Plan!

"The Lord delights in the way of the man whose steps He has made firm; though he stumble, he will not fall, for the Lord upholds him with His hand" (Psalm 37:23-24).

WEEK TWELVE
Day 1

Date

"I have finally accomplished my weight loss goal. I have tried for over thirty years to lose weight never to quite reach my goal. With the spiritual and emotional support from *Weigh to Win* and Lynn Hill, I have finally lost over seventy pounds. I know the continued support is there for me to maintain my weight loss. Thank God for *Weigh to Win.*"
—Peggy

_____

_____

_____

_____

_____

_____

_____

_____

Day 2

Even the woodpecker owes his success to the fact that he uses his head and keeps pecking away until he finishes the job he has started.

_____

_____

_____

_____

_____

_____

_____

_____

_____

_____

Day 3

"Praise be to the Lord, my Rock, who trains my hands for war, my fingers for battle. He is my loving God and my fortress, my stronghold and my deliverer, my shield in whom I take refuge" **(Psalm 144:1-2).**

_____

_____

_____

_____

_____

_____

_____

_____

_____

_____

Day 4

Not everything that is faced can be changed, but nothing can be changed until it is faced.

_____

_____

_____

_____

_____

_____

_____

_____

_____

_____

Day 5

"The Lord is faithful to all His promises and loving toward all He has made. The Lord upholds all those who fall and lifts up all who are bowed down.

"The eyes of all look to You, and You give them their food at the proper time. You open Your hand and satisfy the desires of every living thing" (Psalm 145:13-16).

_____

_____

_____

_____

_____

_____

_____

_____

_____

Day 6

The way to acquire enthusiasm is to believe in what you are doing and in yourself, and to want to get something definite accomplished.

_____

_____

_____

_____

_____

_____

_____

_____

_____

_____

Day 7

_____
Date

"For I know the plans I have for you," declares the Lord, "plans to prosper you and not to harm you, plans to give you hope and a future" (Jeremiah 29:11).

_____

_____

_____

_____

_____

_____

_____

_____

_____

_____

Dear Friend in Christ,

I used to be reluctant to take my children to the amusement park because most parks had those awful turnstiles. I was afraid that I would not make it through or be embarrassed by having to turn sideways and squeeze my way in.

Shortly after reaching my weight loss goal, I traveled to Seattle. While visiting one of the city's famous tourist spots, I looked ahead to see my "horror of horrors"—a turnstile. All the old fears came over me like a wave. I stopped and paused for what seemed an eternity when a voice from within spoke to my trembling spirit and said, "No, Lynn, you can walk on through. Your new body will fit easily through that turnstile. I am so proud of you. Walk on in victory, dear one, walk on." From that time on I began to see myself as the trimmer, healthier person I had become.

> *"May He give you the desire of your heart and make all your plans succeed. We will shout for joy when you are victorious and will lift up our banners in the name of our God" (Psalm 20:4-5).*

Day 1

_____
Date

Do not confuse wishes with wants. When you want *something, you go out and get it. When you merely* wish *for something, you just wait for it to come to you.*

_____

_____

_____

_____

_____

_____

_____

_____

_____

_____

Day 2

_____
Date

"Folly delights a man who lacks judgment, but a man of understanding keeps a straight course" (Proverbs 15:21).

_____

_____

_____

_____

_____

_____

_____

_____

_____

_____

_____

_____

Day 3

_____
Date

"Pessimism never won any battle."
— *Dwight D. Eisenhower*

_____

_____

_____

_____

_____

_____

_____

_____

_____

_____

_____

Day 4

_____
Date

"I am the light of the world. Whoever follows Me will never walk in darkness, but will have the light of life" (John 8:12).

_____

_____

_____

_____

_____

_____

_____

_____

_____

_____

Day 5

_____
Date

True confidence comes from our ability to uncover and accept our weaknesses and to discover and use our strengths.

_____

_____

_____

_____

_____

_____

_____

_____

_____

_____

_____

Day 6

_____
Date

Taste makes waist.

_____

_____

_____

_____

_____

_____

_____

_____

_____

_____

Day 7

_____
Date

"Success, success to you, and success to those who help you, for your God will help you" (1 Chronicles 12:18).

_____

_____

_____

_____

_____

_____

_____

_____

_____

_____

_____

Weigh to Win, Inc.
113 E. Washington
Suite 108
Plymouth, Indiana 46563
1-800-642-THIN

To purchase the Weigh to Win
Weight Management System,
please visit your local
Christian bookstore.